DANIELLE FREY

To the Edge and Back

A Memoir of Mental Illness

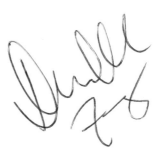

For Twyla,
May you always have the courage to be yourself.

Contents

Introduction

Before writing this book, I was confronted about my illness by someone who intended to out me and discredit me. In the moment and for days afterward, I kept replaying the words in my head, "Is it true that you have bipolar disorder?" The words stung and made my whole body numb with anxiety. At that moment, I chose to be truthful and confirmed in front of a group that I did have bipolar disorder. I suspect that the person who outed me half expected me to lie, but I remained true to myself. Until that happened, I could count on one hand the number of people outside my family who knew about my illness. I felt betrayed that this person had brought up such personal information about me. I thought that the people around me would question my character because of my medical condition. Fortunately, this wasn't the case. I was disappointed that someone would try to use my illness against me. That experience has given me the courage to share my story. Mental illness is nothing to be ashamed of. To the Edge and Back is a story about learning to live with bipolar disorder that I hope will inspire others. I lived in a deep depression for nearly a decade before taking a trip that changed my life forever. Since then, I've lived another decade in control of my illness with excellent stability and support. Until recently, I've kept my story to myself, fearing the stigma I would face. However, the desire to share my experience is overwhelming. Whether you are a new mom experiencing postpartum depression or someone with a mental illness like me, I hope you will enjoy reading my story and take comfort in the fact that you are not alone.

I

Part One

"If you know someone who tries to drown their sorrows, you might tell them sorrows know how to swim."— H. Jackson Brown Jr.

1

Running on a Wheel

On a sunny spring day in June 2012, I found myself cruising through the canals of Venice, Italy. Not on the slender boat of a gondolier but a yellow and red speed boat with the word "Ambulanza" written on the hull. I was escorted from my hotel through the narrow alleyways to the nearby vessel by two handsome dark-haired men. I was wearing a multi-coloured plaid dress, a pair of black velvet heels, and a wicker bucket hat that covered my bright red pixie hair. The air was salty and heavy with the musty smell of the surrounding lagoon. The boat cut through the blue-green water with force and purpose. The lines between fantasy and reality were beginning to blur. My mind was playing tricks on me. Worst of all, none of my friends or family knew where I was going.

What I will never forget is where I ended up.

***

I was excited to travel overseas for the first time. I had been slowly packing and repacking my giant, red backpack for weeks. I had planned a detailed itinerary with accommodation, transport, and activity options like touring the Colosseum in Rome and the Louvre in Paris. Although I was planning to travel on a budget, staying in youth hostels and travelling by rail, this trip was the most expensive thing I'd ever paid for besides tuition. I had saved up for nearly a year to be able to afford the trip, and I had been looking forward to it for just as long. Some days, I would daydream about sitting in a piazza or discovering art in a museum. Whenever I was having a bad day, I would think to myself; soon you'll be in Europe exploring the world! The excitement of this trip and the university applications I had recently mailed out were the only things motivating me and giving me hope.

I was twenty-four and living in a four-story walk-up apartment with an ugly brown exterior. When I first moved in, my cat caught a mouse and brought it to me as a treasured gift. I chose to live by myself, not because I could afford it, but mostly out of stubbornness. I had recently graduated from college, earning a Bachelor's Degree in Sociology, making me the first in my immediate family to earn a degree. My dad worked as an industrial refrigeration mechanic, and my mom worked in various healthcare positions. My parents had two children, of which I was the oldest. Although she was four years younger than me, my little sister, Victoria, was always someone I looked up to. She was wise beyond her years, and I often asked her for advice. During tough times, she was the glue that held our family together.

I didn't attend a big university but participated in a smaller community college. I grew up in a rural Albertan town, and the thought of attending a large university campus in the big city was intimidating. I was just seventeen when I left home to start my studies, and like many teenagers, I couldn't wait to get some freedom.

Attending a smaller school didn't make it any easier to graduate. I worked part-time, and it took me six years to finish my degree. I loved being away from my narrow-minded hometown. Sociology was appealing to me because I was fascinated with counterculture and wanted to challenge the status quo by learning all that I could about society. Going to college was a way out, but I admit I hadn't chosen a practical field of study or given much thought to what I might do afterward. Rather than move back in with my parents, I was determined to make it myself.

I was lucky to work at the local public library as a student page while finishing my degree. After I graduated, I worked three part-time jobs including two separate positions at my college library in addition to my public library position. As a page, I listened to music on my iPod while sorting carts of materials and putting the books back on the shelves. I loved working at the library and knew early on that it was where I wanted to spend my time. The library was this utopian space where anyone could borrow to their heart's content. I enjoyed the quiet atmosphere and respected the library's order. It gave me the sense of safety and stability that I was missing in my life.

When I wasn't working or studying, I devoted most of my spare time to playing roller derby. I had joined a league a few years prior. We had games once every few months and trained vigorously two to three times a week. Our games, or bouts as we called them, were a spectacle only eclipsed by our epic after-parties. Roller derby is a demanding sport that appeals to a specific niche of people. Usually, people who are a bit punk rock with something to prove. I found great camaraderie among this unique group of women, and it's where I met my derby wife, Taran. A wife in roller derby is a term of endearment given to your best friend on the team. She and I became great friends on and off the derby track.

Staying busy with work and roller derby gave me an energy that was addicting. My body was constantly in motion, and my mind was forever spinning. Life felt chaotic at times, and it was hard to wind down and sleep at the end of the day. I often turned to alcohol to relax, and it wasn't uncommon for me to consume a bottle of wine a night. I used alcohol to self-medicate. I had started drinking alcohol in my early teens as an act of rebellion. As a college student, drinking made me forget my financial troubles. I had many drunken adventures that, while fun at first, soon became less dazzling.

I had become caught up in a cycle of responsibility and recklessness between work and partying. I started to feel burnt out from working, and the partying started to lose the level of escapism that it had offered before. I found myself feeling confused and hopeless. I was all alone and felt lost. What was I going to do with my life? Would I be working part-time jobs forever, or would I find myself a fulfilling career?

When I thought about my future as a millennial, "follow your bliss" came to mind. I suppose that meant to be passionate about what you choose to do in life. I questioned what I was passionate about. Although I had gained a few years of experience working in libraries, there were only so many jobs that I could apply to. I would need further education to pursue more advanced positions. My parents always instilled in me the value of education while growing up. I learned that it could be my ticket to a better life.

Having just finished school with a pile of debt, I was wary about going back again so soon. At the same time, I didn't see that I had any other choice. I decided to attend graduate school and study library science to become a librarian. I gathered my application letters from previous teachers and coughed up the application fees to three separate schools. Although my grades were never top of the class, and I was hesitant that I would get accepted, I had no other option. It was libraries or bust.

While I waited to hear back from schools about the fall, I focused on the upcoming trip to Europe. I was going to be travelling with Taran. She was a skilled roller derby blocker and a gifted painter studying fine art at college. Although not a proclaimed goth, the aesthetic appealed to her since most of her wardrobe was either black or gray-toned. Her signature haircut with bangs constantly changed colours from purple to bright red or turquoise. Like me, she was short, but what she lacked in size, she made up in personality. She could draw attention wherever she went. Taran and I spent almost every day together leading up to the trip. We were inseparable until she left for England a few weeks earlier to explore the continent with her boyfriend. Following their journey together, she and I had planned to meet in England and continue travelling just the two of us.

Despite the excitement of my upcoming travels, I was not happy most of the time. My mood was consistently low, and I would cry often. One evening I sat on the bathroom floor and felt like a wave of darkness was devouring my whole body. It felt like I had fallen into a deep well and had no way of crawling back out. My self-confidence had seemed to evaporate over the last few months. I was unsure of myself and my future. A few weeks before leaving for my trip, I decided to talk to my doctor about my mental health.

I sat on the narrow table inside the examination room at the doctor's office, trying not to crease the thin paper underneath. The doctor entered and greeted me warmly. I was nervous. She

7

asked me a few questions and then gave me a prescription that I reluctantly accepted.

Following the appointment, I sat in my car and felt like an absolute failure. I cried and thought about how pathetic my life was. The fact that I needed antidepressants felt like such an overwhelming personal weakness. I collected myself, looked in the rear-view mirror, and saw my bloodshot eyes reflected at me. I started to tear up again. There's something about seeing yourself cry that makes you unable to stop. I drove home quietly, contemplating my life. When I arrived home, I opened a bottle of wine like I had done so many other nights.

2

The Big Three

My parents and I gathered in the departures section of the Calgary International Airport. My red backpack, complete with a Canada flag luggage tag, was packed, and I was ready to go, but my parents were reluctant to see me leave. It was my first time travelling solo. They were apprehensive. My mom, a lifelong catholic, gave me some religious keepsakes to take with me on my journey; a cross and a pendant of St. Christopher, the patron saint of travellers.

My mom is the tallest person in my immediate family. As a plus-sized woman, she often outweighed my dad. She spent most of her adult life wanting to be smaller. She never completed any advanced education and worked primarily in healthcare. Over the years, she performed some odd jobs, including a blackjack casino dealer and a school bus driver. She did what was needed to support her family, including being a stay-at-home mom when my sister and I were too young to be at school. She liked celebrity news and small-town gossip.

As a girl, I always marvelled at her extensive makeup collection. She wanted to feel beautiful and had many lotions and potions to assist with this. She wore her hair long and blonde. When we were growing up, my sister and I weren't allowed to cut our hair. Our parents had us keep it long and blonde, just like moms. When I was a teen, I came home with it clipped to my shoulders and dyed dark purple. My parents were furious. I managed to keep it that way for a few months.

"Don't worry," I reassured them, "everything will be okay." We said our goodbyes and I boarded my transatlantic flight to London, England. It was the longest flight I had ever taken. I found it difficult to get rest. My excitement and the confines of travelling in economy made it difficult to sleep on the nearly nine-hour flight.

Once we landed at the Gatwick Airport, I found a payphone and used my calling card to notify my parents that I had made it in one piece. I met my friend and her beau inside the terminal, and we made our way by train to our hotel. We stayed together in London and explored Brighton beach the next day before heading back to the airport to fly to Italy. We planned to do the big three, Rome, Florence, and Venice, then make our way through Austria to Germany and France, then back to England.

After a quick three-hour flight, we arrived at Rome's bustling Leonardo da Vinci International Airport. We sat at the back of the plane next to the toilets, but we were fortunate to be one of the first people loaded off the aircraft as they deplaned through the front and rear doors. We walked down the attached stairwell onto the cement below. The air was warm with the smell of fuel. The airport was about half an hour from the city of Rome, so we arranged for transport via shuttle van to take us to our hostel.

The van driver was a short, cute, older man who hardly spoke English. He threw our backpacks in the back of his white passenger van while we got settled into our seats with the other travellers. We sat closest to the front. The van driver was surprisingly aggressive behind the wheel despite his small stature. He drove with one hand on the steering wheel. The other hand hovered above the horn. Ready to strike at any moment. He weaved in and out of the lanes at high speeds. We arrived at our hostel without incident.

We stayed at a backpacker's hostel located along a narrow alleyway not far from the Termini train station. When we walked through the two enormous wooden doors, we were greeted by fellow travellers and friendly staff. We got the keys to our six-person female dorm and walked up the three flights of stairs to get to our room. Having never spent a summer away at camp, I had never experienced staying in shared accommodation before and didn't know what to expect. The room did not seem large enough to fit two people, let alone six.

My friend chose the bottom bunk, and I took the top in between two magnificent windows. The time change, the jet lag, and the awkward dormitory bunk beds made it challenging to sleep those first few nights in Rome. My thoughts were racing. I kept thinking about all of the fun things we would experience, about all the possibilities. I was distracted by the party downstairs. While Taran slept, I stayed up all night in the hostel bar, listening to music and playing drinking games with the other travellers. We partied until the church bells rang out in the early morning hours.

I tried to check my emails and maintain contact with my family at least once a day. There were a few computers at the hostel that I could use and an internet café down the street to make long-distance calls. While checking my email, I found something important waiting for me. It was a message from Western University congratulating me on my recent acceptance into their master's program. I was thrilled, overjoyed, ecstatic! Not long before, I had received two rejection letters from two other schools I had applied to, and my hope was running out. Upon receiving the news, I rushed to the café to call my parents. I wept with joy, which I had rarely done in my life. My family was excited, and they congratulated me. Having their support meant the world.

I learned that a fellow Canadian woman staying in our dormitory lived in London, Ontario which was the location of my university. When I told her of my recent acceptance to Western, we exchanged information, and she offered to show me around once I had moved. My life had taken a turn for the better. I suddenly felt enlivened with hope and happiness. I was having so much fun that I decided to stay an extra night in Rome while my friend moved on to Florence.

It was pretty late when I eventually arrived in Florence. I immediately became lost. I tried to find an internet café to get my bearings and send a message to Taran. I found internet access, but I was distracted by funny videos on YouTube. I laughed and laughed hysterically. One of the other customers complained about me. A worker asked me to leave. I managed to find another hostel to stay at, but it had a strict curfew. I got locked out that night.

I wandered the streets, wondering where I would stay. I came across a man who appeared homeless. As I approached him on the road, he held something out in his hand. It was a tiny copper wire that he had bent beautifully into a small pendant. I offered him a few Euros. It then dawned on me that I was just like him at that moment. I had nowhere to go.

I was troubled. I kept moving through the streets on my own. I went to a hotel lobby to get warm and take a seat. I ended up meeting a local man who worked at the hotel. I explained to him that I was locked out of my hostel, and he offered to let me stay at his apartment. He was very tall with broad features, and he spoke English reasonably well. We drank red wine and had great conversations late into the night. The encounter was wholly platonic, and I'm grateful for the kindness this stranger showed to me. After a great evening, I fell asleep on a cot near the window.

I woke up the following morning to a cacophony of noise outside. The apartment was located near the Mercato Centrale, a famous market in Florence. Vendors had started to set up for the day, and people began to flock to the area. Not wanting to overstay my welcome, I thanked him and left at an early hour.

Taran and I eventually connected online and made plans to meet at the train station the following day. We had pre-booked the next leg of our journey. If I made it to the train station on time, I knew I would reunite with my travelling partner on our way to Venice. In the meantime, I decided to enjoy my time alone in Florence.

I visited the exquisitely sculpted statue of David at the Accademia Gallery. There were hearts carved into his eyes. Afterward, I stumbled into a British pub and drank some pints. I wrote my name up on the wall using a permanent marker. I chain-smoked cigarettes and drank caffe freddo's outside the carousel at the Piazza Della Repubblica.

When we met at the train station, Taran was not pleased. I had arrived five minutes before the train departed, and she was worried that we would miss each other again. When I arrived on the train, I was wearing an oversize white t-shirt with red wine stains down the front. We were sitting next to an Italian businessman and his wife, and Taran was embarrassed by my dishevelled appearance. My speech was pressured. I had difficulty communicating. I kept going on about how I could speak Italian, describing it as a "miracle." I convinced myself that I had picked up a second language in days.

I wanted to practice my new skills with the businessman sitting beside me. I turned to the man and started blabbering in English with the odd Italian word thrown in. I asked the man if he could understand me. He nodded his head up and down with a sympathetic "Yes." I turned to my friend. "See!" I exclaimed to Taran. She kicked me under the table to get me to shut up.

The journey to Venice was tense and awkward as I tried to explain what had happened. We arrived in the ancient city and found our accommodation. This time a three-star hotel located in a quiet square across from an 18th-century church. We got settled into our room, and I changed my outfit, then we ventured out to eat. We found a quaint restaurant and had a pleasant meal together. She told me about the tour she had taken through Tuscany. After our dinner, we started walking back to the hotel when I began to try and speak Italian again.

I was speaking English to the world, but it was fluent Italian in my mind. Taran was becoming extremely frustrated with my uncharacteristic behaviour. It wasn't long before we had a falling out. We ended up arguing right on the street in front of a crowd of tourists. We decided it would be best for her to return to England and be with her boyfriend. She gathered her things at the hotel, and I walked her to the train station. We said our goodbyes amicably.

Although I had maintained contact with my family when I first arrived in Italy, it became harder to communicate when I got to Venice. Luckily, there was a payphone not far from the hotel. I used my calling card to phone home, but there was no answer.

I left a message for my family. My mom said she knew by my voice that something wasn't right.

Following the fight with Taran, I started acting strangely. I was emotionally upset and had a strong desire to go to a church. I had not been to church in several years. I paid a gondolier fifty Euros to take me to a church. I didn't realize that churches were everywhere in Italy, so our canal journey was not long. The gondolier walked me inside. I walked to the front of the church and placed my hand on the alter. My behaviour got me some attention. I demanded to speak to a priest. The priest did not speak English very well, and he seemed agitated by my presence.

When I got back to the hotel, I took a very long, scorching shower. I marvelled at the sensation of water dripping onto my skin. Every pore on my body felt like it was dancing. I was hypersensitive to the feeling of the falling water. I thought that I was turning into a demi-god. I left the shower and put on my plaid dress and wicker bucket hat.

After some time alone in the room, I began taking all of the items out of my backpack. I was looking for things to build a shrine on the window sill. In my delusion, I wanted to start a new religion. I placed mundane objects very carefully together as if they held some sacred significance.

I began to hear voices, not just any voices. I listened to the voices of the dead.

I heard my grandmother, who had passed away when I was fourteen, and a childhood friend who had died earlier that year. I started to scream upon hearing their voices so clearly in my head. I screamed so loud that the hotel staff came upstairs to check on me. I braced myself against the door with all of my might so that they couldn't get in. I continued to scream. Someone called emergency services, and the first-responders arrived to take me away. I demanded a pair of sunglasses to go outside before leaving with them. A woman working at the hotel gave me a pair of hers. Everything was so beautiful as we stepped outside.

3

Meeting the Boss

I felt like a celebrity getting an escort to a private boat. In my mind, I was going to visit the pope about the new religion that I was going to make. I didn't know that I was being taken to the Venice hospital's psychiatric ward.

When they admitted me to the hospital, I showed them my passport and gave them a handwritten note that I had prepared before my trip. On the piece of paper was my mom's contact information. Not long after being admitted to the hospital, I became aware that I was in a place I couldn't leave. I started waving my Canadian passport around, insisting that they let me out. I complained that it was illegal to keep me there against my will. I completely lost my temper and screamed at the nurses. I swiftly knocked a pile of magazines off the table onto the floor.

As the days passed, I began to enjoy my stay in the hospital. A cat lovingly referred to as the Boss lived at the nurse's station. There were separate wings for men and women. I shared a room with another woman. She kept trying to take my things. It was her stuff, to begin with, that I had taken as my own. I made friends with a man in his thirties. The ward had a lovely outdoor courtyard where we could get some sunshine and smoke. I had taken up smoking a few days earlier and didn't always finish my cigarettes. I gave my leftover tobacco to my new friend for him to finish. Smoking outside was a simple pleasure that I looked forward to.

Being manic was such a frightening yet euphoric experience. Everything was so vivid and alive. The timeless European architecture took my breath away. Everywhere I went felt like a dream. While I was manic, I experienced what it's like to be free of all convention and societal constraints. I lived in my reality with no comprehension of the social norms typically expected of me. I had difficulty communicating, and I felt very alone. I couldn't control my emotions. One minute I was crying tears the next minute, I was laughing out loud. I experienced a decreased need for sleep, delusions of grandeur, hyper religiosity, and my mind was in complete chaos.

As I was eating my Caprese salad for lunch, the nurse informed me that I had a visitor. She took me to the doctor's office, where Taran and my mom greeted me. I was surprised to see Taran, but I knew that my mom would find her way to me.

My mother and I didn't have the best relationship while growing up. Her mother, whose voice I had hallucinated, had passed away from cancer when I was coming of age. Although my mother and I were both grieving her loss, we became disconnected from one another. I started to rebel and drink while my mother became deeply depressed. Despite our strained relationship, I never doubted that my mother cared for me and loved me. I was fortunate to have her there with me in Italy. I will always be grateful that she came to find me.

Once she arrived in England, Taran had contacted my mom on Facebook to let her know what had happened. When my mom called my hotel, they informed her that they had to call emergency services and that I was no longer there. My dad contacted the Canadian consulate, and they confirmed that I was still in Italy. With the help of her family, my mom was able to book a flight to London the next day. She met up with Taran, and they flew to Venice. They collected my things from the hotel then ventured to the Venice hospital, where they worked with the doctors to get me discharged. The process took a few days, but I was finally released. I was not well. My parents worried about flying home commercially, and they contemplated using a mediflight to transport me home. Although I was not yet stable, my mom and I flew home to Calgary on Air Canada.

Upon landing in Calgary, my dad and my younger sister greeted us. I was wearing mismatched clothing provided by the hospital in Venice. My family was glad to have me back, but they were deeply concerned about my well-being. I went to my parent's house, and they took care of me while I worked to recover. There was no psychiatrist in my parent's town, so I attended telehealth appointments. I received an official diagnosis of bipolar 1 disorder.

At first, my family and I were all shocked and confused. My parents assumed that I had experienced a breakdown caused by stress. It was hard for them to accept that their daughter had a chronic mental illness. From the time I received my diagnosis, I did all that I could to educate myself about the disorder. I trusted the medical advice I had received. I was compliant with my new medications even though they had horrible side effects.

The medicine they put me on in Italy was not available yet in Canada. Early on, I was over-medicated on Risperidone, an antipsychotic. My eyes rolled back into my head, and my tongue stuck out. I didn't leave my parent's house for a few weeks. My family worried that I was never going to be the same. As the summer weeks passed, I began to make progress. My psychiatrist adjusted my medications, and I started to resemble myself again. Soon, it was time for me to return to work and go back to my apartment. My parents drove me back to my city to regain some level of normalcy.

One night while brushing my teeth, I thought I saw someone standing behind me in the mirror. I freaked out and called my parents. After thoroughly checking my apartment and confirming that no one was there, I still couldn't calm down. I called my doctor and said that I had seen someone in my apartment. Knowing my recent history, he advised me to go to the hospital. I drove there, and they admitted me to the E.R.

Unlike the other patients waiting, they put me in a room with a door. They strapped my arms to the side of the bed. They discharged me a few hours later, thank God. It was an indication that I was not yet stable on my new medications. I ended up having to quit my jobs. I wondered how I would be able to attend graduate school in the fall, but I knew that it was something I had to do. It was awful timing to have had a manic episode that summer. I was determined not to let my new diagnosis stop me.

II

Part Two

"We cannot change the cards we are dealt, just how we play the hand."
—Randy Pausch

4

Heading East

G rowing up, the fall was such an exciting time in my life that I always looked forward to. After spending so many years as a student, the fall signified the beginning of another school year and an opportunity for a fresh start. As the days gradually got colder, summer began to end, and I began to feel that special feeling of anticipation once more. I packed up the items from my apartment and moved them into storage at my parent's house. I had never lived outside of Alberta, but soon, London, Ontario would be my new home. I was limited in what I could bring since I would be flying across the country. I packed only the essential items like my laptop, school supplies, and clothing which I stuffed into two oversize suitcases.

My mom flew with me to Ontario to help me get settled into my new living arrangements. She rented a car and helped me purchase a new twin bed and mattress. I was grateful to have her help. I rented a room in a house with two younger undergraduates and a graduate student my age who was studying anatomy. I got along well with my older roommate, but the two young roommates liked to party. It was a massive distraction while I worked to recover and focus on school. When I mentioned that I had bipolar disorder to my roommates, one commented, "Oh, I heard that can be cured; just take some vitamins." After one semester, I found a different place to live.

The people in the next household were more mature and very supportive of my situation. They knew I needed to take medications daily and needed a quiet, stable space. I stayed in that house for the remainder of my degree. When I wasn't working on assignments, I enjoyed cooking or watching hockey with my one roommate, Greg. He had a Golden Labrador, which he let me take out for walks. Another roommate had a cat. After having to re-home my cat before leaving Alberta, it was a great comfort to have pets around the house. I was glad to be no longer living all alone. Throughout my studies, I lived with several other students. The roommates in this new house were some of the best people I could have asked for. Their support was essential in my recovery since my friends and family were not nearby. My roommates were there for me when I needed someone to talk to, and they helped make life as a student more enjoyable.

After being diagnosed with bipolar 1 disorder, my life began to feel like a balancing act, as if I were walking along a thin tightrope. Whether it was my moods, behaviour, or medications, it felt as though I could lose it all with one slight slip. I had to be very careful about what I said or did. Tell the wrong person about my condition, and I risked losing new friends, as had happened when I started graduate school. Stay up too late or have too much to drink, and I would risk having a horrible mood swing the next day. Go away for the weekend without my medications, and I could risk ending up back in the emergency room.

As I learned more about my illness, I began to build up healthy habits and identify what things would trigger me or set me off balance. One of my main focuses was sleep. My doctors always stressed the importance of getting enough sleep. I knew that I could go manic if I were to become too sleep-deprived. This was a constant worry of mine. While I was first figuring everything out, I was over-medicated. I would sleep for ten or more hours a night. I experienced horrible grogginess that felt like having a hangover but without the drinking. With the help of my university doctor, I was able to adjust my medications so that I could sleep an average amount of time.

Earlier in my recovery, I had to relearn how to feel and express my emotions. I constrained myself not to feel too happy because it reminded me too much of what it felt like to be manic. The trauma of experiencing mania frightened me. I was afraid to let my mood get too elevated again. I tried to be less excitable and more even keel. As months passed, I became more comfortable expressing stronger emotions and allowed myself to feel joyous once more.

I was incredibly fortunate to receive psychotherapy from my psychiatrist while attending university. Therapy can be costly, and without my student benefits, I would not have been able to afford it. I will never forget my university psychiatrist for how he helped me recover following my episode. He helped me come to terms with my diagnosis and break down the stigma by educating me about the disorder.

While I was a student, Margaret Trudeau came to speak at my university. She also had bipolar disorder, so I decided to hear her talk. Mrs. Trudeau spoke about her past adventures, like partying with Mick Jagger of the Rolling Stones. She shared how she had to work hard every day to manage her bipolar disorder. She maintained her stability through medications, eating a healthy diet, and exercising. I thought it was remarkable that mental illness could affect anyone, no matter their social status or wealth. Her story was inspiring to me, and I admired her courage.

It took me sixteen months to complete my master's degree. Although I struggled to complete assignments at first, my confidence and abilities grew with each semester that passed. By the end of my studies, I excelled academically. I was finally starting to feel like myself again but the best version of myself. I was no longer using alcohol to cope. I had built up my self-care strategies, and I had learned how to take care of my health. I left Ontario with a clear and open mind, ready to start the next portion of my life.

5

My Missing Piece

After finishing graduate school, with no job prospects and no money, I had no choice but to move back in with my parents. They were happy to have me home. I was glad that I would always have a place with them should I need it. Like many new graduates, I relentlessly began my work search and sent out a slew of applications. While waiting to hear back from my prospective employers, I began volunteering at local non-profits. I taught myself how to knit and created an online dating profile to see who may be out there. I met the man I would later marry.

He lived in a city about an hour from my parents. He was getting ready to move 500 kilometers away after accepting a new job offer in Edmonton. My mom had a dentist appointment in the city that he lived in, so I took the opportunity to go with her and meet up with my online crush.

He was born a world away in Sri Lanka during a civil war, two years before I was born in Canada. Somehow, we ended up in the same country, then at the same school, just missing each other by a few years. By the time I had enrolled and moved halfway across the country, he had graduated and moved to my home province. Had I finished my sociology degree a little earlier, we could have met in Ontario at graduate school. Instead, we were both in Alberta, meeting an hour from where I grew up. I do believe that it was some level of fate that brought us together.

We met at a local coffee shop close to the river. It had been years since I went on a date, even something as casual as coffee. I arrived first and ordered an iced coffee. My date came as I waited anxiously in the pickup line. I went up to him in line and introduced myself. "Hi" he said, "I'm Rajees." He was handsome, with beautiful brown skin and dark hair. I hoped that he couldn't tell how nervous I was. He grabbed his drink then we went outside to sit on the sidewalk patio.

One reason that we had connected online was that we were both in the same field. When I found out that he was a librarian, I was thrilled. I knew couples who had gotten together in graduate school, and I was always jealous of their shared bond. I thought it would be simpler to date another librarian. They would be able to understand my profoundly misrepresented line of work.

We sipped our drinks and joked about all the beautiful people at our school. As a student, I always felt surrounded by young people much more attractive than me. I always felt intimidated to approach anyone romantically. I thought it was a good sign that he could relate. We finished our drinks but stayed much longer, sitting outside and talking in the sun. Rajees kept laughing and smiling at all my remarks. I'm sure we could have stayed there chatting all afternoon, but it was time for me to pick up my mom from her appointment. We walked together to our cars, and he asked me if I liked sushi. I replied "Yes!" enthusiastically. We parted ways with plans for a second date the following night.

Despite not knowing him very well, I disclosed that I had bipolar disorder on our next date. I was pretty reluctant to share my diagnosis with most people. Still, I immediately trusted him enough to share my secret. He acted like it was no big deal and reassured me that it didn't change his feelings about me. Rajees wasn't like other men I had dated in the past. He was an intellectual. Our conversations challenged me and made me think about the world. I found that incredibly attractive. We had a lovely second date which led to a third, then a fourth before he had to move away.

After he moved, I accepted my first job working as a librarian in Rocky Mountain House. We dated long-distance for a year, then I moved into his tiny downtown Edmonton apartment. Living together was a natural fit. We enjoyed going to restaurants and exploring the city. After a few years of saving, we bought our first home. It was a new infill home located in one of Edmonton's oldest neighborhoods just north of the city center. After five years of dating, we decided to get married. Rajees proposed to me privately at our house.

Our wedding was a small ceremony held on top of the high-level bridge inside a historic streetcar. As the streetcar perched atop the narrow bridge, my eyes darted to the windows, and I saw how high up we were. My stomach did flips. I couldn't tell if my nerves were from the heights or because I was about to be married. Committing to one person for your entire life is a giant leap of faith. We took that leap together on the streetcar and chose one another as companions. With Rajees by my side, the ride seemed a little less scary.

Rajees became an excellent source of stability in my life. That's not to say we were boring. We had lots of fun adventures together. We travelled to cities around the world, including New

York and Beijing. We went hiking in the Rocky Mountains and attended live concerts together. He was a consistent source of love in my life that allowed me to grow as a person and flourish into a strong, competent woman. Without his love and support, I would not have been able to tame my mental illness for so many years.

Shortly after getting married, we began the discussion of starting a family. I hadn't always wanted to have kids, but I began to picture us together as parents. We had rescued a cat. When I saw his affection towards her, I knew that someday he'd be a great dad.

6

TTC

I began to contemplate whether I should have kids, given my medical condition. I knew there was a risk of postpartum psychosis, but I thought it couldn't happen to me. I wondered if it would be ethical to have a child knowing they may also struggle with mental health as I had for most of my adolescence. I thought about how many of those with bipolar disorder die by suicide. My university psychiatrist once told me that future children could inherit several medical conditions, such as high cholesterol. Since it is treatable, he suggested it would be no worse to inherit bipolar disorder. He said I shouldn't let that possibility stop me from having kids. Besides, if my future children were to get bipolar disorder, I would be well equipped to help them cope and manage their illness.

Beyond the moral dilemma of whether we ought to have children, I faced the physical challenge of needing to adjust my medications. Valproate, the anti-epileptic drug that I took to stabilize my mood, had been shown to have teratogenic effects. I needed to stop taking medicine to have the best chance at a healthy pregnancy. The drug had worked so well to keep my

31

moods stable for several years, so I hesitated to go off it. I didn't know how I would fare emotionally off of the medication. What if I had another episode? Would I be able to function well at work? Would Rajees still love the person I was without a prescription? I worked with my psychiatrist to wean off the Valproate despite these concerns. We agreed that the risks were too high to go completely un-medicated, so I started an antipsychotic with less chance of causing congenital disabilities. It took a few months to get my medications successfully switched.

Soon after stopping Valproate, my anxiety went up. I couldn't cope with the stress as I had before. My psychiatrist put me on the anti-anxiety medication Buspirone. Despite going off the Valproate, there was still a risk that my new medicines could cause congenital disabilities. The possible side effects were hard to accept. Together, Rajees and I determined that my risks were more significant than the low risks to a developing fetus. Although I knew the chances were now much lower, that there was any risk made me feel incredibly guilty. I wished that I could have gone medication-free. It was my psychiatrist's job to prescribe medications to keep me stable. I willingly went off a drug that had worked so well for me for many years. I appreciate that my doctor listened to me and accommodated my desire to have children. I was fortunate to have a relatively predictable and steady home life that afforded me the luxury of stopping my medication.

Rajees and I travelled to Honolulu, Hawaii, for our honeymoon. I was stable on my new medications by then, so we casually started trying for kids. We tried this approach for approximately six months until March 2020, when the COVID-19 pandemic was announced. I will never forget that week in March when I was collecting groceries. I entered the store and encountered masses of panicked shoppers scrounging to grab items from the newly stripped shelves. That's when I realized that the coronavirus everyone had been talking about was a real threat. They say that in a fire, people panic and often grab random items. That day at the store, I panic purchased two giant bags of dry lentils fueled by my need to prepare. The pandemic made everything stand still. We didn't know how bad it would get, so people panicked and expected the worse.

We were both fortunate to keep our jobs and work remotely; however, the pressures of the pandemic made it difficult to keep trying to conceive. The world as we knew it had changed entirely. We had no idea how things were going to work out. The atmosphere made us question once more whether we ought to have kids. With all of the stress and uncertainty, it was an easy decision. We would pause trying to conceive until things had calmed down.

Months later, things started to brighten at home and around the world. There was a glimmer of hope as normalcy seemed to return. That was when we doubled down on our efforts to have children. We planned with conviction. We used apps, recorded my basal body temperature each morning, and used ovulation test strips to predict the perfect opportunity. Over and over, we were met with a negative result each month. I was not prepared for the emotional ups and downs that came with trying to conceive. Each month I held my breath and crossed my fingers that this would be the time that worked out. Then, I'd have to wait an entire two weeks to see if we were successful or not. As a young woman in my twenties, I used to be relieved to get my monthly period but while trying to conceive, getting my period meant another failure.

In the fall of 2020, we found out that Victoria and her husband were expecting. The news was gut-wrenching to hear since, to my knowledge, she didn't even want to have kids. She was my only sibling, and I loved her dearly. I couldn't help but be happy for her. She and her husband came over to our house while my parents visited. I had purchased a cake decorated with baby pink and blue to share the news with our mom and dad. My mom squealed with excitement and looked at me encouragingly upon seeing the cake. Then I said, "No, it's not me." Then she looked at my sister and was in disbelief. It was a great moment that I'll never forget, and I'm glad we could share it. I told my family that we would become parents when the time was right.

I took an early pregnancy test approximately four weeks later, and a faint double line appeared. I ran down the stairs to meet Rajees and confusingly said, "I think we might be pregnant." He shrieked, "What? What are you sure?". I told him it was still very early and that no, I wasn't sure. We waited anxiously for the next few days until the date when my period was due. The date came and passed. We retested again. This time, two lines were visible, revealing that we were, in fact, pregnant! After all the heartache and tedium of trying, we were finally successful. We embraced each other as I wiped away happy tears.

7

A New Life

Throughout my pregnancy, I had stayed on medication and had been relatively stable. I suffered from nausea and vomiting, but it was never severe enough to warrant hospitalization. I'm not sure why it's called morning sickness because, in my experience, nausea and vomiting can happen at any point during the day. I would often finish a meal only to run to the bathroom to expel the contents I had just consumed. My doctor prescribed me medication to help manage the sickness, but it did little to help.

I was about thirty weeks pregnant when my obstetrician diagnosed me with gestational hypertension. I had never had problems with my blood pressure before, so this new condition came as a surprise. I had to complete blood work and have my urine tested every week leading up to delivery. They screened me for preeclampsia, a potentially dangerous condition that pregnant women can develop. My doctor prescribed medication to help regulate my blood pressure. Even with medication, my blood pressure increased the closer I got to full term.

Around my thirty-eighth week of pregnancy, my doctor

advised me that it would be best for my health and my baby's health to be induced two weeks ahead of my due date. I agreed and signed the paperwork. They gave me instructions to go to the hospital that weekend. I was nervous about being induced but excited that the long pregnancy would soon be over.

We arrived at the hospital on Saturday morning to begin the induction process. The doctors did an internal exam to check my cervix. They found that I was not dilated or effaced, so they gave me a vaginal suppository to ripen my cervix and initiate the induction. They sent us home and said to come back the following day by noon. We came home and tried to relax before the inevitable labour that was about to come.

Later that night, I drew myself a bubble bath and sat in the tub, patting my big belly. I spoke to my daughter, "I'm so excited to meet you," I told her. In the back of my mind, I was dreading the pain of giving birth. I thought to myself, relax, you're about to become a mother, which is something beautiful you should be proud of. I exhaled and felt a sense of peace. Rajees and I went to bed that night excited and full of uncertainty.

Around four in the morning, I woke up to use the bathroom, something I had done numerous times throughout the end of my pregnancy. This time something felt different. I felt a gush of liquid escape between my legs as I walked down the hall. Luckily for me, I had been prepared and was wearing an adult diaper just for this very situation. I went to the toilet, and more liquid gushed out. I knew from my prenatal classes that this was amniotic fluid and that my waters had started to break. The nurses informed us to come back to the hospital sooner if my water broke. I was reluctant to go back because I had envisioned myself labouring at home to start. We decided to get a few more hours of rest at home and then return to the hospital around seven that morning.

I didn't realize that the rhythmic contractions would start soon after my water had broken. At first, they felt like light menstrual cramps, but they were noticeable and uncomfortable when we returned to the hospital. As we waited in the triage bed, the contractions became more robust, and I felt intense pain. I moaned out loud in discomfort. I was frustrated that we had to wait to get admitted because I thought I had progressed much further than I had. When the doctors checked my cervix, I was only one centimeter dilated on Sunday morning.

Since my water had broken and the contractions were getting stronger, they admitted me to a labour room for monitoring. I laboured in that room using nitrous oxide gas. At one point, I hopped into the shower to get some relief. After three or four hours, they offered me morphine as the pain ramped up. A gush of amniotic fluid escaped with every bounce of my birthing ball and every contraction. The pain was excruciating, but it was productive. Unlike most pain caused by injury or illness, this pain had an end goal in sight, empowering me. My contractions continued for several hours. I continued, contracting and gushing shamelessly. After twenty-two hours of labour, I finally received an epidural. As my lower body started to numb, the pain began to subside.

At one point, I threw up. The hospital required that I get tested for COVID-19. A nurse came into my room completely covered with a gown, gloves, face shield, and a mask. I was anxious to get tested because of the long nose swab. I wondered if it would hurt. She plunged the giant swab into my nose. "That's it?" I asked. We were all done. When you're in labour, everything else that may cause you discomfort seems inconsequential. We were officially placed on COVID protocol while waiting for the test results. Due to the protocol, every person entering our room had to wear complete P.P.E.

During my labour, I had been awake for almost twenty-four hours. I was able to get a few hours of rest after receiving the epidural. When I awoke, my whole body started to shake. I thought maybe I was in the transition phase of labour when the cervix dilated the last few centimeters. I was rechecked. The goal was to get to ten centimeters. I was still only at one centimeter after labouring for an entire day.

My heart sank as I looked over at Rajees and started to cry. All I wanted was to meet the little girl who I had talked to in the bathtub the night before, but things were not progressing as they should. A kind nurse came over and reassured me that we would meet our baby one way or another. We had not planned to have a cesarean section but Rajees and I agreed that it was the most likely outcome.

I continued contracting until early Monday morning. A group of doctors came in to see me. They advised me that we needed to get the baby out soon since it had been over twenty-four hours since my waters broke. Both the baby and I had elevated heart rates. The team of doctors and nurses moved with urgency, and I became aware that this situation had become emergent. I could not continue labouring on my own. They suggested that I undergo surgery. The nurses brought in a gown and scrubs for Rajees to change into. I laughed as he put the gown on backward, and I asked one of the nurses to help him out. The nurses wheeled my bed out of the room, and I met more surgical team members in the hallway. The journey to the operating room felt so surreal. I started to get anxious as we passed through the elevator and rushed by different parts of the hospital.

When we arrived in the operating room, there was a group of

at least ten people, each focused on preparing for the surgery ahead. The medical team moved me to a narrow operating table. Then, they spread my arms onto two tables on either side. My eyes teared as I gazed up at the bright lights overhead. This was the moment I had been waiting for. Finally, it wouldn't be long before I could meet my baby girl. Soon I would hear her high-pitched cry and see her tiny face, something I had imagined for a long time.

As they continued to prep me, I noticed that I could feel the cold iodine on my stomach and feel the sharp pricks of the testing needle on my skin below. The anesthesiologist prepared me with oxygen to put me under general anesthesia. Internally, I started to panic, but I remained calm for everyone preparing to operate. I knew that Rajees wouldn't be permitted in the room if they put me under anesthesia. "Tell my husband what's going on," I yelled frantically. Not long after, I was passed a mask and asked to inhale deeply. The last words I heard were, "You might remember this." Moments later, our little girl was born without her mom and dad to greet her. I will always be eternally grateful for the medical team who brought my daughter safely into this world.

Following the surgery, I woke up in a panic. I was in a bed with people on either side of me pushing me through the hallway. "Where was my baby?" I wondered. When I didn't see or hear her, my chest tightened up, and I started coughing for air. "Ativan," I gasped, and the doctor agreed to administer the benzodiazepine. They placed the drug underneath my tongue and rolled me into the surgical recovery unit. I started to calm down.

As the nurses checked me and I began to come to, I noticed a figure in my peripheral vision. I was annoyed that they had let someone into my recovery unit. Then, I turned my head and realized it was Rajees, and he was holding our daughter. I cried out a sigh of relief. He brought her over to me and asked, "Do you want to hold her?". I was still waiting for the anesthetic to wear off, so I declined. She was beautiful and healthy with a mound of thick brown hair and big brown eyes like her dad. They wheeled me up to our room after the nurses finished checking me. We stayed in the hospital for two more days. I will never know how we made it through the first night with our girl. The whole thing felt like such a blur.

I tried to sleep as much as I could so that my body could recover, but more importantly, so my mind could rest. I had stayed up for almost twenty-seven hours before being put to sleep during surgery. I went without my psychiatric medications during labour, and I knew that if I didn't get more sleep before leaving the hospital, I would risk going manic.

As we adjusted to becoming parents, I knew that I was in a very precarious position with my mental health. Before leaving the hospital, I asked a nurse to talk to a psychiatrist. They seemed reluctant and explained that only those admitted to the psychiatric ward could talk to the psychiatrists. I called my usual psychiatrist and set up a phone appointment for the following week. By the time I spoke with her, I was already starting to adjust my medications to keep up with my changing needs. Although I tried to get ahead of things, I was heading towards mania. In the weeks that followed, I slept no longer than two hours at once and I went back to the emergency room three times.

III

Part Three

"Out of all the things I have lost, I miss my mind the most."
— Mark Twain

8

The Unraveling

The drive home from the hospital with my newborn daughter was one of my most anxious experiences. I was so scared that someone would hit us, injuring our precious cargo. We had to stop at the drug store to get my pain medication. Rajees went in while I sat in the front seat with the doors locked. The air conditioning was blasting cold air since my daughter was born in the middle of an unprecedented heatwave. The shrill sound of the air conditioner started to mimic the sound of a baby crying. I turned back to check on my daughter. She was okay. Was I hallucinating, or was this just new parent anxiety?

Soon Rajees came back with my prescriptions, and we went home. Before leaving the hospital, we had called my mom, who was two hours away, and asked if she would come to help us. We had not planned to have visitors so soon because we wanted to figure out our routine as a new family. Since I had unexpectedly undergone surgery, we thought we could use the extra help. My mom showed up ten minutes after we arrived home, leaving us little time to experience what it would be like just the three of us.

Although I was happy to have her there, friction started to build between my mom and my husband. Following the surgery, my mobility was limited. I couldn't move up or down the stairs very quickly. The surgery confined me to the top level of our house for one week. We expected my mom to help us keep things clean and assist with meals since I couldn't go downstairs. She helped to take care of the baby during the day. While it was nice, it was not what we truly needed help with.

Our newborn demanded to be fed and changed every one to two hours. Although I had tried pumping after my surgery, my milk supply never came in. Not being able to breastfeed my daughter hurt me in ways I never realized it would. Just as my body had failed to progress during labour, my body had been unable to provide for her. I felt like I was less of a woman because I couldn't do this seemingly natural task. I knew this was ridiculous but I couldn't help but feel let down.

We had no choice but to formula feed our daughter. By the time we prepped a bottle, fed the bottle, and changed her, it was nearly time for us to do it all over again. It was exhausting work, especially at night. Rajees and I devised a plan to share the nights so that one of us could get some rest every other night.

One evening, I took the night shift in the nursery and started to feel pain in my lower back. I woke my mom up to give me a hand. I told her my back was hurting, so she suggested I try laying down in her bed. As I lay down, the pain in my back became worse and worse. I had a previous tailbone injury, and I wondered if it had become inflamed during my labour. I took a heavy dose of Tylenol to cope with the pain. The pain wouldn't subside, so I woke Rajees up, and we decided to go to the hospital.

When we arrived at the hospital, I could hardly walk, so they pushed me to the emergency room in a wheelchair. I lay on the emergency room bed writhing in pain. The doctors checked me, but they couldn't find the source of the pain. They offered me opioids, but I declined. I called for a nurse, and she offered to adjust my bed to make me more comfortable. She sat me up at a different angle and adjusted my legs that had been hanging off of the bed.

My pain instantly disappeared. Rajees was in disbelief. I had gone from crying in pain to virtually good as new with a simple adjustment. The doctors came back in and seemed perplexed. I was discharged and walked out of the emergency room feeling like a new woman. We were confused, but we were relieved that my pain was gone. We theorized that I had experienced psychosomatic pain caused by stress. We hailed an Uber to go home. As we stood outside waiting, a feeling of peace rolled over us. We were going to be okay.

When we arrived home, our newfound sense of peace shattered. We were sitting in the living room when my mom stood up from her seat. She handed over the baby and said she wanted to talk to us. She stood up and began pacing around the room. She was very agitated and asked us bitterly, "Why am I even here?".

Throughout the week she had spent with us, she had tried to offer us advice, but we had done our research and wanted to do things differently. My mom took a lot of pride in raising two children, and she was offended that we wouldn't take her advice. She raised her voice as she started to ascend the stairs. She continued yelling at us from her perch on the stairwell, telling us that we shouldn't read books and that we were doing it all wrong.

We sat calmly on the couch below, but our fight or flight response had kicked in. Rajees, who was holding our daughter, stood up in a motion to protect his family. My mom suddenly stormed up the stairs and slammed the door to her room. Moments later, she returned and left the house, slamming the front door behind her. We were shocked. We felt disrespected and unsafe in our home.

We decided it was time for her to go home. We called my dad and told him what had happened. Usually, my dad can calm my mom down when she gets upset. We wanted him to let her know she was no longer welcome in our home. She returned to pack her things and left quickly without looking at us. As the door finally closed behind her, I started to sob uncontrollably.

Losing this social support left me vulnerable while I was already recovering. This time in our lives was supposed to be full of happiness. Instead, I had experienced tremendous pain, seemingly out of nowhere. Now I had experienced a falling out with my mother. I reluctantly blocked my mom's phone number. I turned my focus towards taking care of my baby while trying not to think about what had transpired between us.

I felt increasingly disappointed that we didn't have a home full of people to congratulate us on the arrival of our baby. I had the urge to invite everyone I knew over to our house because I wanted them to share our happiness. Perhaps I was trying to fill the void created when my mother left us. It's normal to receive visitors from well-wishers after the arrival of a baby. The pandemic changed that for us. Our daughter was born during a time of social isolation, and I was sad that more people couldn't come to see us.

It had been a week since we left the hospital, and we were starting to enjoy our new family. I moved up and down the stairs by this time, although I was still exhausted and weak. Neither of us had been getting much sleep, and we knew we still needed some help. We contacted my husband's youngest sister in Ontario and asked if she would fly out to Alberta to help us. She was a nursing student and had a summer job administering vaccines during the pandemic. At first, she was reluctant to come out because she didn't want to leave her summer job; she needed the money for school. We offered to pay for my sister-in-law's flight and pay for missing the last few weeks of work. She took a few days to think it over.

While we waited to hear back from my husband's sister, we went back to our system of sharing the nights. I sat with my daughter in the middle of the night in the nursery. When I looked up at the doorway, my vision had started to blur. I saw two doors before me. After leaving the hospital, the nurses who came to do our wellness checks instructed me to monitor my blood pressure. If it got above 160/90, they advised me to go back to the hospital. I assumed they were worried about me developing postpartum preeclampsia. Blurry vision can be a symptom of that condition, so I decided to take a blood pressure reading with the cuff I had used during my pregnancy. It was high; 150/88. I woke Rajees up and explained that my blood pressure was high and I had blurry vision.

I started to freak out and felt an impending sense of doom. I asked him to go down to the pantry and grab as many snacks as possible. He returned, and I ravenously ate the food he brought back. I started to chug a water bottle that was on the night table. Rajees tried to calm me down and said It was just a panic attack. He offered me an Ativan, and I screamed at him, "Do not give me an Ativan!". I convinced myself that I was crashing and would die if he gave me a sedative.

We called the health link number for new parents. They advised us to contact the emergency number 911. With a pit in my stomach, I called 911 and gave them my information. Soon, help was on the way. Two burly paramedics arrived at our house and stood staring calmly at me as I lay in our bed. I was holding a pillow behind my neck, convinced that if I let my head fall back, I would fall asleep and never wake up. One of the men took his kit and measured my blood pressure. It was now in the 190s. They asked if I wanted to see a doctor, and I shouted, "YES!". After taking a moment to get dressed, I walked arm and arm with one of the paramedics down the stairs to the waiting ambulance outside. I kissed my husband goodbye, unsure of when I would be back.

When I arrived at the hospital, there was quite a long wait to get into an E.R. bed. They gave me a temporary bed and wheeled me into the hallway. I felt absolutely exhausted and wanted desperately to sleep. I was afraid that if I closed my eyes, it would be for the last time. I missed my daughter terribly, and I kept looking at pictures I had of her on my phone. It was hard to be all alone, separated from my family.

When I finally saw the doctor, they retook my blood pressure. The number had gone back down, and the doctor ruled out postpartum preeclampsia. I explained my fear to the doctor that my blood pressure would get so high and "poof" just like that; I would die. He assured me that's not how high blood pressure worked. He explained it to me like redlining a car. If you rev your engine too high, it won't explode, but its performance will suffer over time. This analogy reassured me. I was given another prescription for blood pressure medication and told to follow up with my family doctor.

After being discharged, I waited outside for my ride when I finally looked down at what I was wearing. On the bottom was a pair of black and pink pajama pants with a Victorian-era print.

A white and black polka-dotted nightdress was on the top with an orange cardigan sweater. I laughed to myself because none of it matched, and it looked as though I had just come from the psychiatric ward. I thought about how I must have looked to others and continued to laugh.

After I left him, Rajees called his sister crying and explained what had happened with my mom and that I was back in the hospital. She knew we were not well and agreed to come and help us. She quit her job and flew out within a day.

9

A Bowl Full of Cherries

We were so happy when my husband's sister arrived. Her young spirit and bubbly personality brought us much-needed comfort and joy. She was enamoured with our daughter and took great care of her. She switched with us and took every other night shift. While she was with us, I started acting strangely.

Instead of sleeping, I stayed up late on my computer one evening. I thought we were getting cyber-attacked and had to update all of my important passwords. I found a password generator online and auto-generated 100 character passwords to be extra cautious. I felt like I could communicate with the technology in the room, and I imagined that the t.v turned on by itself to send me a message. I questioned whether I was even a human. I thought I might be a humanoid Cylon like in our favourite T.V. show Battlestar Galactica.

I hid my delusions from Rajees and his sister. He was confused about my high energy levels since he knew I had not been sleeping much, but he assumed it was okay as long as I was productive. It wasn't until our daughter's two-week appointment that he realized I was not well. He noticed that I kept trying to talk to everybody while we were out in public, but I had difficulty getting my words out. He tried to ask the doctor about giving me something to sleep, but I reassured him I was okay.

Rajees was concerned that I wasn't sleeping enough, so he tried to stay with me until I could get some rest. I remember trying to sleep down in the basement, but I had to get everything just right. I had a unique wedge-shaped pillow to angle my upper body, along with earplugs and eye patches. I closed my eyes and tossed for a few minutes. My exhausted body desperately craved sleep, but my mind was terrified to let go. The darkness scared me, and I fought the feelings of fatigue.

After trying for a few minutes, I threw off my eye patches and said I needed one more thing. That's when my husband's patience ran out, and he ran upstairs. "I just need one more thing, and then I'll sleep!" I yelled at him, but he was already gone. I ran after him, but he didn't want to see me. He kept trying to keep me out of our bedroom. I could tell he was on the phone with someone, so I went in and grabbed the phone. "Who is this?" I asked rudely. The woman on the other end said she was with 911. At first, I was confused; why had Rajees called 911? Then I was relieved because he was anxious, and maybe the paramedics could help him calm down. I went downstairs to wait for the emergency services to arrive.

My phone rang. My husband's best friend and his wife were calling to see how we were doing. I told them Rajees was not acting like himself and that help was on the way. As I talked to them, I sat on a stool with my head poking out of the front door waiting for help to arrive. Rajees was sitting at the top of the stairs looking down at me. I took the phone up the stairs to him, and we took turns talking to our concerned friends on the other

51

end. In my mind, Rajees was just a nervous new parent, and he needed to calm down. As I sat there waiting, it felt as if time had slowed to a complete crawl.

Finally, two female police officers and two paramedics arrived, one of whom was at our house a few nights before. "I knew you'd come back!" I exclaimed as I walked out the door to greet everyone. The officers had their hands cautiously on their waistbands but soon relaxed when I started to talk to them. We entered through the open door, and I tried to explain the situation. One officer and one paramedic went upstairs while the others stayed with me in the kitchen. I was so glad to have them there because Rajees wasn't well. I offered them coffee, but they declined.

I chatted with the female officer and discovered that we shared the same first name. Soon the other officer came down to join us in the kitchen. She commented about how clean and organized our home was. She motioned to the bowl of cherries sitting on the kitchen island and complimented me for putting out a smaller bowl just for the pits. I looked at the bowl full of cherries in front of me. I was so delirious that I didn't even realize that's what I had done. To the outside I appeared organized and put together but internally, my mind was falling apart. One paramedic asked me about the extensive board game collection, specifically which one was my favorite. I started to ramble on about our favorite game and an online version that he could play for free. I had loads of energy, and I was happy to have visitors in our house.

The police officers tried to persuade me to go to the hospital to get checked out. They said that my husband was worried about me and wanted me to go in with them. "Go back to the hospital again?" I thought. I had been there twice since delivering my baby, and the thought of going back a third time seemed incomprehensible. But since I was worried about my husbands' well-being and loved him very much, I agreed to go back to the hospital with the police. Before leaving with them, I needed to change my clothes and collect the particular items that made me feel safe. They didn't want me to go upstairs, so one of the officers went up to grab my things. After about three trips up and down our stairs, the officer returned with everything I would need to go back to the hospital. She had gathered a dress, shorts, and a small sentimental jewelry box with a lucky coin and gemstone inside.

The three of us walked to the police vehicle, and they opened the back seat for me. The police officers were very kind, and we had a pleasant conversation together. While we were driving to the hospital, I had a terrifying thought that the world was ending. The officers waited with me in the hospital waiting room until the hospital admitted me to the emergency room. They said it was very nice to meet me and wished me well.

10

The Ward

I was in the emergency room for three days while waiting for an inpatient bed in the psychiatric ward. During this period, my mental state started to deteriorate even further. I had delusions that it was the end of the world and that I embodied Jesus coming to save those around me. I imagined that those around me in the hospital needed my help. I was harmless, but my presence agitated some patients.

Two nurses grabbed me on each arm. They forced me into a room with one window that looked out into the hallway and locked the door. They usually put violent or aggressive patients in this room. The nurses put me there because I wanted to help others. I was furious that they locked me inside. I started to unhook the flimsy mattress from the hospital bed to throw it. The nurses wheeled the bed away, leaving me the mattress. I refused to sleep on it and instead slept on the floor two weeks after having major abdominal surgery. I woke up sometime later in excruciating discomfort. "Ahh!" I screamed out in pain. The nurses came in and helped me up off of the floor. They finally let me out of the locked room and into another room with a curtain.

Rajees came to visit me at my request but soon after he arrived, I realized that it was a mistake. He was nothing but caring towards me, but I was upset that he wouldn't partake in my delusional reality. I asked him to leave and told the nurses not to let him come back. This decision was devastating to him. My sister and mom came to see me while in the emergency room. I could tell they were worried, so I tried to put them at ease by singing and dancing, as I had done to help my fellow patients. I kept a white notebook that I used to scribble mad ideas in. On one page, I had a list of professions that I wanted to try once I was released; among them, of course, was a psychiatrist.

For a brief period, I almost forgot about my daughter completely. It was as if she never existed even though I carried her for nine months and laboured for over twenty-four hours so that she could be born. I felt so tormented by the delusions that my regular life stopped making sense. That's what's so scary about psychosis. Your whole world and everything you care about can disappear. Luckily for me, I didn't lose anything or anyone permanently. I came back.

The hospital psychiatrists certified me twice and admitted me to the hospital's top-floor psychiatric ward. I referred to it as the penthouse. I was lucky enough to have a room all to myself. There were no other women there my age. Most of the patients I interacted with were much older, and it appeared that they had been there for quite some time. The dining room was converted into a common room, equipped with an old laptop attached to a flat-screen T.V. Patients took the opportunity to listen to their favorite songs on YouTube. For the most part, two older female patients controlled the laptop. The women played Neil Diamond's *Sweet Caroline* on a loop.

There was one computer in a separate room closest to the

nurses' station. The computer room is where I spent most of my time when I wasn't resting in my hospital bed. I checked my emails and played games online. One day I decided to make a playlist. At first, the list had twenty songs, then fifty, then one hundred. I kept adding pieces until the playtime totaled twenty-four hours. Song after song, I found hidden meanings and connections to the lyrics. The music helped keep my spirits up in an otherwise dull place.

In the weeks following my daughter's birth, I spent money. I purchased random items online like a napkin holder, a team-building game, and a Franz Kafka book. After I became hospitalized, I continued to buy things online. I placed an online grocery order and got it delivered to our house. I believed that I could communicate with my family at home by sending them items I had purchased online. Rajees disabled my credit card. I used his credit card to buy an $875 lottery ticket. Fortunately, he was able to get the charge reversed.

To help pass the time, I began doing the exercises posted on the walls around the circular hospital unit. I walked laps around the unit until I had reached multiple kilometers each day. The food in the hospital was adequate. While staying in the ward, I suddenly changed my diet to become a lacto-ovo vegetarian. I lost twenty-five pounds four weeks after giving birth with my constant movement and my new diet. After about a week in the ward, the Doctors gave me privileges to leave for thirty minutes and come back, but I had to stay on the hospital grounds. I explored the hospital, looking at the art that adorned each floor, and admired the many plants living inside.

One day while in the elevator, I came across a young couple. They each were wearing tags that had NICU written on them across their chests. I asked if they had just had a baby, and the woman got teary and said, "Yes, we are going to visit her right now. She's in the NICU". I smiled and congratulated them, and they seemed so happy that someone had recognized them as new parents. Meanwhile, I was a new parent myself, but I didn't dare tell them so. I couldn't explain that I was separated from my baby because of my mind.

I received excellent care and compassion from my team of nurses. I was surprised by how young the nursing staff were. Most were around my age and I gravitated toward them. I had a phone call with Rajees one day that upset me. My nurse came in to the room as I started to cry. He asked me why I was upset, and I told him that I had just had an argument with my husband. It was hard to be away from my family, and I wanted Rajees to see me and bring our daughter. He said that he wasn't ready yet. My nurse assured me that I was doing the right thing by being away from my family while I focused on getting better. He said that I was working to recover and doing a good job. It was comforting to have someone listen to me and encourage me.

Unlike many of my fellow patients, I was fortunate to have visitors come and see me while I was in the hospital. Although we had a falling out, my mom returned to the city. She stayed in a hotel so that she could come and see me almost daily. Even my Boss came to see me. She was a great listener, and it meant a lot to have her there. My dad eventually came to see me, and so did Rajees.

At first, I was disappointed that Rajees had not come to see me sooner. He had his hands full caring for our daughter, and understandably, he felt hurt by what I had said to him while in the emergency room. When he did visit, he brought our daughter with him to the delight of all of the nurses. We took some photos and shared a tender moment together as a family. It wasn't the ideal location, but in my hospital room, the world was starting to feel right again.

Rajees came back to the hospital on his own to attend sessions with my psychiatrist. They had wanted to put me on Lithium, and I was apprehensive since I'd never taken the drug. I was reluctant to go back on the Valproate to stabilize my mood even though it had kept me sane for many years before getting pregnant. With encouragement from Rajees and my medical team, I agreed to start taking the Valproate once more. Although my family knew I needed to restart the Valproate, I had to be the one to decide to begin retaking my medication. I found it very difficult to make decisions about my treatment while still ill. With each day that passed, my mania started to subside, and it became clearer what I needed to do to go home and be with my daughter.

As my condition improved, I was granted a day pass and eventually a weekend pass to go home and see my family. By this time, my husband's family had come to visit, and it was overwhelming at times to be around everyone. Going back to the hospital was bittersweet because I didn't want to leave my daughter, but I knew I wasn't strong enough to be at home. I needed to return to the ward and work on my recovery.

Rajees dropped me off at the front entrance to the hospital. After he drove away, I walked to the front doors but discovered that they were locked. I started to get anxious because I had to be back at the ward in ten short minutes. Another patient who was using a walker approached the doors. She was finishing up a smoke. "Come with me," she said confidently, "I know the way." She explained that we had to enter through the emergency room doors in the evenings, which were located on the east side of the hospital. We walked together and chatted along the way

58

about what we were in the hospital for. I told her I had just had a baby but needed some time to work on myself. As we rounded the corner to the E.R., we came across a group of smokers. I was apprehensive as we approached the group because they looked a little intimidating from a distance. As we got closer to the group, I began to recognize familiar faces. It was some patients from the ward. I smiled warmly. "Welcome back," one of them said to me.

I stayed for about two weeks altogether before I felt confident enough to return home. I was sad to be away from my daughter knowing that I had missed weeks of her life. Ultimately, I was proud of myself for taking the time that I needed to get healthy once more.

IV

Part Four

"Never to suffer would never to have been blessed."
— *Edgar Allan Poe*

11

Putting in the Reps

We lost certain things to the pandemic; a loss of normalcy, opportunities to travel, and our sense of time. We also gained a new family member and a new respect for one another. We gained a better understanding of my chronic illness. My husband and I gained renewed care for the vows of our marriage that kept us together during trying times.

Before trying to conceive, Rajees and I had a pretty comfortable life. We stuck to our daily routines and faced very few challenges. I knew that having a child someday would be a huge obstacle for us and I was excited about the opportunity to grow as individuals. Learning to be a good parent for my daughter was the biggest challenge I faced since recovering from Italy several years before. It took over a year to fully recover from my first manic episode.

In contrast, it took me a lot less time to recover following my second psychotic break. After being released from the psychiatric ward, I met with my regular psychiatrist in her office. She couldn't believe that it had only been a day since my release.

She kept asking me, "And you got out yesterday?".

I needed to find stability quickly after being released from the hospital so I could care for my daughter. My husband's vacation time would end soon, and I would quickly become the primary caregiver. It helped that I resumed the Valproate medication that I went off of to become pregnant. I had significant social support. I had visitors come to see me in the hospital and follow up with me when I got home. I worked hard to show up each day for my daughter. Caring for her was like an exercise. With each change and each feeding, I put in the reps to get stronger so that she would be healthy and taken care of.

When I first came home from the psychiatric ward, I was unsure of my ability to care for our daughter. I couldn't do so many reps. I got tired quickly and was overwhelmed. I had always envisioned that caring for my baby would come naturally to me, but now I felt out of place. I lacked the confidence and the physical stamina needed to care for a newborn. I was awkward holding her during feedings, and I struggled to complete her never-ending diaper changes. Rajees confided in me that he wasn't sure I could handle everything.

Despite my insecurities, each day, I pushed through. Most days, I felt exhausted. Following my release, my mood was low, and I experienced a mild depression. It was inevitable to feel depressed following the mania; after all, what goes up must come down. In addition to my low mood, I was struggling emotionally. I didn't feel the same happiness that I had felt shortly after the birth. I found it challenging to find joy in my new reality as a mom. I was disappointed with myself. I felt as though my mental illness had robbed me of the opportunity to get to know my baby in those first few crucial weeks. I was grieving the loss of a typical postpartum experience.

I learned to hang on to the tender moments as a new mom. I wasn't always happy, but I felt glimpses of it now and then. The foggy depression started to lift as I continued to put in the reps and build my daily routine. I began to enjoy spending time with my daughter instead of dreading getting out of bed every morning. Our bond grew stronger with each day that passed, and so too did my confidence. Having the support of my family and friends was crucial during this time. They reminded me that I could do it and believed in my abilities even if I did not.

When my daughter was six weeks old, I finally forced myself out of the house to join a mom's group meeting for a walk in the park. I had only been out of the hospital for a few weeks, and I wasn't quite feeling like myself, but I pushed through my apprehension. It was the first time I had driven myself anywhere in nearly two months. I stopped driving near the end of my pregnancy and could not drive while I recovered from surgery. It felt great to have some independence back, but I had trouble connecting with the other moms. I felt as though I had been through hell and back. It was hard to relate to the problems that others were experiencing. How could I tell people I struggled with depression after experiencing psychosis a few weeks earlier? Although I didn't open up to the group about my situation, I enjoyed being outside and socializing. I kept going to the group each week and found that the routine was beneficial. It gave me something to look forward to each week and helped build my confidence in venturing out with a newborn.

I learned that postpartum psychosis (P.P.P.) occurs in about 1-2 women per 1000 deliveries. With over a million people living in Edmonton, I wondered how many other women had experienced what I had after giving birth? I wanted desperately to connect with these other women, to share our stories and experiences.

Soon after being released from the hospital, I stumbled upon an online support group for P.P.P Survivors.

I hadn't thought about myself as a survivor before. I believed that the designation of survivor was meant for those who had experienced some near-death experience. I hadn't been close to death, but my situation could have become a lot worse without medical intervention. P.P.P. is a medical emergency that requires immediate attention. I could have harmed myself or others unintentionally. I am so fortunate that I got the help that I needed. I'm amazed by my husband's bravery and the love he showed when he made the call to 911. He was patient with me and remained calm even though it was one of the most challenging moments of our relationship. As it turned out, I was a survivor after all. I came back from a very dark place and with the support of those around me, I got better.

Finally, I could connect with others who shared a similar experience. Most of the group's members lived in the United States. Some of the mothers were months and years into their postpartum journeys. It had only been a few weeks since everything had happened to me. It was refreshing to meet these women and see how they recovered after experiencing postpartum psychosis. Other survivors had started blogs. One mom had started a walking campaign to raise awareness and funds. Some women went on to have additional children without experiencing further episodes. Their stories brought me a little bit of hope.

When I thought about our family, I always envisioned having two children. During my episode, I experienced hypersexuality and had the great desire to start trying immediately for another child. Even while hospitalized, I was reluctant to restart Valproate treatment again because I was concerned about having another baby. As I started to recover, it became clear that Rajees and I disagreed about having more children. The first month after my daughter was born was arguably the most challenging four weeks of my life and most likely that of my Husband's. His immediate response was that we shouldn't have any more children, but I wasn't so sure. I wanted a second chance at giving birth. I felt like the emergency cesarean birth and the psychotic episode had taken something from me. I yearned desperately to get it back.

Neither my husband nor I witnessed the moment of our daughter's birth. After she was delivered, Rajees was in the hallway outside the operating room. There was a baby in the hallway, and he didn't even know she was his. Having another baby would allow us to have a more typical birth experience. I hoped that by having another child, I would be able to heal some of the trauma I had experienced during those first few weeks.

Postpartum psychosis is more likely to occur in people with a history of bipolar disorder or those who have experienced a previous manic episode. The chances of me experiencing another episode were relatively high. I thought about what we had experienced, Rajees and I, and, although I disagreed with him at first, the thought of putting him through all of it again broke my heart. For my well-being and the health of my marriage, I decided that it was okay to have only one child.

My second episode strained my marriage. My husband had seen a side of me that he had never experienced before. Following my release, I was shaken and emotionally fragile from my experience. We were usually always in tune with one another, but now he viewed me differently. He was cautious about leaving me alone with our daughter. Our mutual trust had been broken inadvertently because of an illness that had slipped out of my control. I felt like it was my fault that I had let it get so bad and experienced psychosis in the first place. I now think that the situation was well beyond my control. What happened wasn't a relapse or a breakdown of my character. It was a medical event that I needed to recover from.

12

A Look Back

I've had a lot of time to think about my first manic episode in Italy. It was a perfect storm that seems almost inevitable now. I had recently started SSRI antidepressant medication, a common trigger for bipolar disorder. I had travelled across time zones, was jet-lagged, and suffered from a lack of sleep. It was spring, and I had travelled to a warmer climate. All of these factors, combined with the excitement of travelling for the first time, helped propel me into mania.

After my first episode, I felt a strong sense of shame and embarrassment for my psychotic behaviour. With time and psychotherapy, I learned how to forgive myself and move on. As I began to heal from the trauma, I kept replaying events repeatedly in my mind. I had a great desire to write. I started a blog to try and piece together fragments of my memories so that I could begin to understand what had happened to me. I had to learn to separate my psychotic behaviour as a symptom of the illness and not a characteristic of who I was. It took me time to process the life-altering experience and I remained unstable for months.

I began to see my illness as a blessing in disguise because I finally got a diagnosis and received treatment. I had lived with depression for nearly a decade since I was a teenager until I was in my mid-twenties. Those years were tumultuous as I self-medicated my moods and energy levels with alcohol. Once I started to receive proper psychiatric care, I felt like I could finally reach my true potential in life. The drugs never took away my creativity. Instead, they helped me to be free. I was no longer hiding underneath the shroud of darkness and depression. The medications helped lift a weight off my chest so I could breathe again.

Years after my diagnosis, my life began to stabilize, and it felt like I was never ill in the first place. My doctors had warned me that this is often the point where many people start to go off of their medications because they think they are cured. I didn't do that. Being compliant with my medications has always been my number one priority in managing my bipolar disorder. While the origins of bipolar disorder and exactly how it affects the brain are not fully understood, medication can manage the condition effectively. Much like how a person with diabetes does not produce enough insulin, people with bipolar disorder may lack certain chemicals in the brain and need medication.

Medication is, of course, not the entire solution. I needed behavioural interventions like living a healthy lifestyle, practicing mindfulness, and using Cognitive Behavioural Therapy, among other things. The same things that keep me physically fit, eating well, getting enough sleep, and exercising help keep me mentally healthy. That's because mental health and physical health are the same. I'm grateful that I've been able to find what works for me both medically and in my everyday life. I try to stick to a routine. I've worked to identify my stressors and eliminate them as much as possible.

Having people who understand and respect your needs is crucial for your mental well-being regardless of whether you have a mental illness. My family has been the central support system over the years, especially my sister, Victoria. While I was going manic after giving birth, she was the one communicating with Rajees and letting him know I wasn't well. Although we had been together for several years, he had only known me while stable. He did not know the signs of mania and didn't realize the severity of the situation.

By the time I had my second episode, I had ten years of experience managing bipolar disorder. I lived each day without fear because I had educated myself about my illness, taken my medications, and worked towards living a stable life. My support system was in place if I should need it.

When I look back at my two episodes, I think about what had changed in the ten years between them. In my first episode, I was travelling and out of my routine. The mania and psychosis seemed to come on a lot faster. The second episode had a slower descent into madness. I was at home for the most part while my mental state started to crumble.

Technology played a more significant role in shaping my delusions ten years later. I convinced myself that the nurses at the hospital were robots and that I may have been a cyborg. I had access to my phone and social media the entire time I was manic and psychotic. I posted some bizarre things to my Facebook page and started messaging many people on Instagram. Luckily, nobody paid much attention, but I feel embarrassed by my need to share my every manic whim on social media.

Both times that I've been manic, I've felt a strong desire to write. The act of writing became increasingly difficult as my mania worsened and the psychosis started to take over. I wanted to write down my rapid flight of ideas so severely, but the connection between my brain and my pen wasn't there. I couldn't clearly express the way I was feeling or thinking. It was incredibly frustrating. Writing this book while healthy has empowered me to express myself in ways I had only dreamed of in the past. Making the conscious choice to share my story with others has been meaningful in my recovery from those traumatic experiences.

I used to view having bipolar disorder as a weakness, my dark secret. As the stigma surrounding mental illness has improved over the last ten years, I've come to view my illness as an asset. I'm not ashamed to have bipolar disorder. It has allowed me to become more reflective as I've worked to identify my triggers and manage my moods. It has given me the ability to be deeply in touch with my emotions and those around me. I've developed emotional intelligence with great practice, allowing me to empathize with others. Over the years, I've learned to be kind to myself and give myself some grace. Healing and recovery have not been linear processes. I've experienced many ups, downs, twists, and turns along the way.

The mind is an exciting thing. It can change how you perceive the world around you and what you believe to be true. My belief in my delusions never faded. I was convinced the world was ending and that I was like a god. I could not be rational and reflective. The only truth that mattered was what I had derived in my head. The experience, while terrifying at times, was also liberating. While not having to follow conventional thinking, my mind was free to explore new ideas. I saw connections in things that I once ignored. My senses became heightened. Just as nature benefits from biodiversity, human society benefits from diverse perspectives and experiences. I hope that those with mental illness will be viewed not for the symptoms of their disorder but by what unique insights they can share with others.

Mental illness can happen to anyone when you least expect it. It is essential to seek out help when you need it, and you shouldn't feel ashamed for doing so. Mental illness doesn't have to define you or become your entire personality. It is something that happens to you, not something that you are. I am not bipolar; I have bipolar disorder. Framing things in this way has helped me accept my identity as someone with a chronic but treatable illness.

I'm still living my life and working to be the best version of myself, not only for me but for my daughter. I know that I will experience further depression and mania throughout my lifetime. I'm not afraid of what the future may bring. I am resilient.

Acknowledgments

Thank you to my sister Victoria for being the glue of my support system and always taking the time to listen. Without your love and encouragement, this book would not have been possible.

I want to thank my loving parents for helping me achieve my dreams. Thank you to my husband for sticking by my side when things were tough and to Pavetha for helping our family when I couldn't be there.

Thank you to the fantastic medical teams at the Royal Alexandra Hospital who delivered my daughter and helped me recover in the psychiatric unit.

Lastly, thank you to the Edmonton community of writers who helped motivate and encourage me.